Psychiatric Evaluation of Children

Psychiatric Evaluation of Children

George Isaac, MD

Writers Club Press

San Jose New York Lincoln Shanghai

Psychiatric Evaluation of Children

Writers Club Press
an imprint of iUniverse.com, Inc.

For information address:
iUniverse.com, Inc.
5220 S 16th, Ste. 200
Lincoln, NE 68512
www.iuniverse.com

ISBN: 0-595-17942-8

Printed in the United States of America

This book is dedicated to all the children and their families from whom I have learned most of what I know of psychiatric evaluation of children.

Contents

Chapter I

Introduction

Psychiatric evaluation of children is the cornerstone on which all treatment efforts for an emotionally distressed, behaviorally troubled, or mentally ill child are built. The capacity for children's psychiatric evaluation stands at a very incomplete stage at present, yearning for research breakthroughs to provide more knowledge on the problems of children. As it stands today, it relies heavily on what can be observed and understood by interpersonal interaction and as such depends almost entirely on the capacity of the clinician to observe, elicit, and understand. The limitations of our perceptive capacities restrict this process almost entirely to the observation and interpretation of the behavior and verbalizations of the child in the context of the history given, with most children today. The ardent hope is that the advancement in technology, especially in molecular biology, genetics, biochemistry, functional brain imaging, and related areas, will soon add dimensions that will make evaluation of children a more scientific and illuminative endeavor, serving as a prelude to more effective if not curative treatment measures. Until such a scenario materializes, we will have to rely mostly on our observational capacities, interpersonal skills, and clinical interpretations to conduct the best evaluation possible in today's circumstances.

Until about the last decade, the published works on child psychiatric evaluations had a strong psychoanalytic bias, a format that does not have significant clinical applications for the type of problems seen in most children today who are brought for psychiatric evaluations and interventions. During the past ten or fifteen years, there has been an appreciable shift to conduct an evaluation that is more in keeping with the expanding knowledge of psychiatric problems in general and to arrive at an internationally acceptable diagnostic understanding and a less speculative formulation. Nevertheless most books or chapters on the psychiatric evaluation of children available today are too vague and scattered in their approach, leaving the student or trainee entering the field somewhat frustrated as to how to conduct an effective, organized, and practical child psychiatric evaluation for clinical purposes. This publication, it is hoped, will at least partially address the need for a brief yet reasonably comprehensive introduction to doing adequate psychiatric evaluations of children.

This publication is primarily intended for the medical student or graduate trainee in psychiatry or child psychiatry and allied fields interested in acquiring the skills to do good, reasonably comprehensive child psychiatric evaluation in a clinical setting.

At least a minimal knowledge of basic child psychiatry and childhood psychopathology is essential to gain full benefit from perusing a publication of this nature. Ideally this publication would be most beneficial in leading a teaching and discussion group by a child psychiatrist, for residents, fellows, medical students, and other graduate-level trainees in child mental health. An experienced clinician could use this publication to full advantage as study and discussion material for trainees and can clarify, critique, and elaborate on the points presented to help develop the understanding and skills of the trainees to become competent evaluators of children.

In this publication the term child is generally used to represent the preschool and elementary school child as well as the adolescent, except where a specific mention is made of the youngster at a particular age group or developmental level to emphasize a point that is unique to that level by referring to the youngster as a preschool child, elementary school child, adolescent, etc.

Chapter II

Points Worth Remembering before Starting the Evaluation

Some Differences Between Evaluation of Children and Adults:

The evaluation of children differs from that of adults in many obvious and not so obvious ways. To start with, almost always a child is brought for the evaluation by the parent, parents, or the guardian because of their concern about the child's behavior, distress, or functioning. Except in an occasional adolescent who may initiate a consultation on his or her own because of personal concerns, the decision to have the psychiatric evaluation is made by the adults, and the child may be a willing or not so willing participant. In all cases the information given by the adults responsible for the child or adolescent plays a crucial role, setting the stage for the evaluation. In the evaluation of adults there are very few occasions, if any, that call for contacting the adult's place of work, even with their permission, to gather ancillary information about them. With children, however, relevant information obtained from their school and teachers would be extremely useful if not crucial in most circumstances.

The use of play is another feature that distinguishes the evaluation of children. The younger the child is, observation of and interaction with the child in play activities often provides information that is difficult to obtain otherwise, such as the activity and energy level of the child, capacity for sustained attention, preoccupations, how they perceive the world around them and crucial figures in their life to be, and capacity for symbolic thinking, to name a few. Play serves as an indirect method by which the child's manner of functioning, concerns, and conflicts could be assessed. This is especially important, as many young children are unable to discuss their concerns and conflicts in a clear and easily discernible manner.

The attitude, stability or instability, personality functioning, awareness, and related factors of the parents play a crucial role in the evaluation and treatment of children, as most information and recommendations regarding the child has to be filtered through the parents, and the parents' influence on the child is crucial one way or another. What information the parent may or may not reveal, what recommendations they will accept or reject (overtly or covertly) etc., play a crucial role in the understanding and treatment of the child. In most child psychiatric evaluations one is dealing with at least three crucial variables: the child and the two parents. At times there are other significant adults, such as grandparents or other extended family members, teachers, and other school authorities who may bring in additional concerns and opinions that influence the evaluation. In the evaluation of an adult unless the adult and the psychiatrist feels there is a strong reason to interview a relative such as a spouse, the evaluation is most often completed by seeing the adult only.

The Child Psychiatric Evaluator

There is a crucial requirement for the child psychiatric evaluator. This requirement is a genuine concern and empathy for the child and parents. Parents and children are often in crisis by the time they are seen in an evaluation. They bring an array of concerns, anxieties, fears, hopes, and despair. There is something unique about the problems and distress of children. In the parental psyche, childhood is the tender period of anticipation and hope for all good things to come. The very suspicion of the development of psychiatric problems at such a tender age sets off an avalanche of emotions in all concerned. The evaluator who is not in tune with these unique concerns and turmoil often comes across as inept or crude in their dealings with the child and family, unaware of the hurts and sensitivities of the people concerned. To obtain the trust of the child and parents in a genuine manner without making false or inappropriate promises is extremely important. Children often will not reveal information that is anxiety provoking or embarrassing to them unless they feel confident that the evaluator is genuinely concerned about their welfare and will only use the information in a sensitive manner to alleviate their distress or rein in their uncontrollable impulses. Adults will often settle for the technical expertise or reputation of a clinician, but it is often not so with children. They seldom "open up" unless they feel they have in front of them a genuinely concerned, friendly, and trustworthy ally.

Good knowledge of children's normal development, delays and deviations that commonly occur in the course of development, and the possible manifestations of various psychiatric disorders at different developmental stages in the cognitively well endowed and the cognitively deficient, are essential prerequisite for conducting a good evaluation.

Flexibility and capacity to improvise during the interview process, depending on the needs of a given situation are the hallmarks of a good evaluator. The psychiatric evaluator of children should be capable of doing a comprehensive evaluation that takes into account the biological, and psychosocial aspects of the child. In today's circumstances a child psychiatrist because of the educational and training background of such a specialist best accomplishes this.

The role of Parents

Psychiatric evaluation of the child is seldom complete without information gathering from and an informal evaluation of the parents or guardian with whom the child is intimately involved in a dependent relationship. In today's world, however, one often sees children who are not living with their parents and the parents may not be available to be interviewed. It is important to get as much information as possible about the parents in all circumstances and to keep in mind that the evaluation is deficient to the degree that such information is lacking about the parents. The biological traits the child inherits from the parents and the crucial role or lack of it the parents play in the child's upbringing and life makes such information vital. This does not in any way, however, imply that childhood psychopathology is caused by parental psychopathology. The relationship is far more subtle and complex. Even if the problem arises primarily from within the child, the dependent intimate relationship the child has with the family often gives the expression of the problem an interpersonal coloring. The distress and/or deviant behavior in a child produces distress and/or deviant behavior in the parents and other family members, which would manifest in a multitude of ways depending on the vulnerabilities of the people concerned. Any treatment recommendation, to be effective, would require the active cooperation of the parents, and so without evaluating the personality structure, likes, and dislikes of the parents, and the presence or absence of major psychopathology in them, one cannot make a treatment recommendation that would be appropriate, acceptable, or likely to succeed. This does not mean that the parents and other family members should be subjected to a formal psychiatric evaluation. How one approaches this issue is discussed further in the "Interviewing of the Parents" section.

The Issue of Time Needed for the Evaluation

Though at times children may have to be seen for the first time in an emergency visit, in general the evaluation should be a pre-arranged affair with the evaluator allotting enough of his or her undisturbed time for the evaluation of the child. On the average this would require a minimum of 2—4 hours in most cases (often posing problems, especially in today's managed care environment). Unless there is a need to implement pharmacological treatment urgently or arrange for in-patient hospitalization immediately (which would require completing an abridged preliminary evaluation quickly to ascertain the immediate needs), it is best to complete the evaluation in two sessions, on separate days, perhaps a few days to a week apart. This gives an opportunity to see the child on two separate occasions, enabling one to observe how consistent or variable the child's functioning and problems are, and also providing a chance to observe the child free of some of the initial anxiety and inhibitions that are common when dealing with a stranger for the first time—and that too in often stressful circumstances. Each session should end in a supportive manner without making false statements or raising false hopes. Allotting enough time is crucial in the evaluation of children. Children are not often very forthcoming, and information is often revealed in bits and pieces of relevant and not so relevant admixtures. Often their statements are vague and even contradictory.

One of the main reasons a child psychiatrist may succeed in doing good evaluations and arriving at clearer understandings when others have failed to do so is because he or she is willing and able to spend enough time with the child and parents in an unhurried manner and gather and review additional information that may be obtainable to arrive at well thought out conclusions. Rushing through a quick evaluation, except in an emergency, is unfair to the child, the family, and the evaluator himself or herself. Once the need for adequate time is explained, most parents are willing to cooperate (though the insurance company may not, which may force some compromises, such as initiating preliminary treatment while obtaining additional information and observational data). In general once an evaluation is started, within a period of two weeks if not earlier, the evaluation should be completed, and the parents and child (in a manner appropriate for the child) should be informed in lay terms what the evaluator thinks the nature of the problem is and what measures could be undertaken to alleviate the problem. In most cases detailed psychological tests and other relevant studies or consultations could be completed later. An exception is a child whose primary problem is cognitive deficiency or a related problem, whose evaluation can be done more efficiently if a psychological test report on the cognitive status is already available.

It should be understood that the diagnostic understanding and formulation arrived upon after the evaluation is only preliminary and tentative. As the child is seen in treatment and as further information and observations become available, some of the understandings may need to be modified, as appropriate. In this sense the initial evaluation of the child has to be followed by a longitudinal evaluation that is on going as long as the child remains in treatment or follow up care. Though this is pertinent for adults also, it is more so for children because the rapid developmental process impacts on their problems and because of the greater uncertainty involved in understanding and interpreting children's behavior and symptomatology.

The Evaluation Report

A child psychiatric evaluation should result in a well-written evaluation report. It is not only essential for present purposes but for future references as well (sometimes even after the child reaches adulthood.) I often find even brief and inadequate reports from the childhood of adult and even elderly patients to be illuminating regarding the type of psychiatric problems they presently suffer from, especially in arriving upon a proper diagnosis. Some pointers on how to organize a good evaluation report are discussed later.

Chapter III

The Evaluation—Part 1

Psychiatric Evaluation of children could be broadly divided into Five Parts:

1. History gathering and interview with parents
2. Interview and observation of the child (including play)
3. Medical/Neurological evaluation of the child, including appropriate laboratory tests, brain imaging studies, and specialist's consultations as indicated
4. Evaluation and interpretation of all data obtained, arriving at diagnoses, case formulation, and the written evaluation report

5. Meeting with the parents and child to explain the findings in lay terms and in a supportive manner, along with discussion of treatment options if indicated.

Of these the history gathering and interview with the parents will be discussed primarily in this chapter. The interview with the child, the mental status examination, and informing the parents and child of the findings and recommendations will be discussed in chapter three.

Starting the Evaluation

In most situations it is better to gather preliminary information from the parents first, so that the evaluator could have a reasonable idea as to the general nature of the problem. An exception would be the case of an adolescent who specifically requests he or she be seen first, either because of the belief that the parents would prejudice the mind of the interviewer by distorting information or because of frank suspiciousness. A usually appropriate format is to see the child and parents together for a brief introductory period initially, followed by interviewing the parents and then the child separately.

Interviewing the Parents

The parents are usually seen together. There are two main goals to accomplish during the interview with the parents. The first is to gather information in detail about the child's presenting problems and symptomatology, as well as past history, family history, developmental history, medical information, and school and social history. The second is an informal evaluation of the parents as people and as parents of the child (including an informal mental status evaluation), and parents' relationship to each other and the child. The informal mental status evaluation is accomplished by observing the relevant processes as parents talk about the child and themselves and by observing their interaction with each other and the child. It is inappropriate and unwise to conduct a formal mental status examination of the parents, though at times even the presence of a major mental illness in a parent may be clearly evident to an experienced observer.

The interviewer should be sensitive to the feelings and concerns of the parents without sacrificing objectivity. The interview is conducted in a supportive manner. By the time a child is brought for psychiatric evaluation, the parents have been going through a mixture of feeling states and experiencing a plethora of emotions: anxiety, fear, depression, hopelessness, guilt, and anger being the more common ones. Even the most seemingly unconcerned of parents blame themselves in some way for having been responsible for the problems of the child. It is wise to keep a few things in mind when interacting with the parents. The first and most important perhaps, is that in most instances of childhood psychopathology, a complex combination and interaction of genetic, constitutional, and environmental factors are at play, and to blame the parents as having been solely or even primarily responsible for the child's problems is extremely naive if not disastrous in most cases. Parents should be viewed as having done what they could, given the totality of circumstances, which include among other things their own genetic make up, emotional vulnerabilities and circumstances in which they live. Very little is accomplished by making the parents feel guiltier. Secondly, it is during the evaluation process that the groundwork for therapeutic interventions and rapport are established, and the best of evaluations is of very little use unless it can be followed by a helpful therapeutic intervention in most clinical situations.

It is better to begin the interview by letting the parents elaborate with the minimum of interventions possible the presenting problem, its development, the course the problem has taken so far, and related issues. At times it may be necessary to guide and refocus the parents if they tend to become too circumstantial or scattered in their verbalizations for one reason or another. As the interview proceeds, points and issues the interviewer feels are important could be brought up, explored, and clarified in detail.

Some important areas to be covered in the interview with the parents:

1. Presenting problem and history of presenting problem

When and how did it manifest; the details of the various aspects and components of them, has it been improving, persisting without change, or is it worsening? What interventions were tried; which ones helped and which ones did not? Ask about specific symptoms and signs that may be pertinent to the particular presenting problem. Ascertain if there was any likely precipitant.

It is very important to ascertain if there is a history of alcohol or drug abuse when evaluating adolescents.

2. Past psychiatric history and treatment history

Has the child had similar or other behavioral or emotional problems in the past? If yes, what was done, and what was the result? Inquire if the problems appeared episodically and, if so, whether the child was well and free of symptoms or problem behaviors between the episodes, or if the symptoms or problems were waxing and waning without periods of full remission.

3. Developmental History

Start with the prenatal history. Explore gently whether the pregnancy was expected or unexpected, wanted or unwanted. (Note that even if the pregnancy was unexpected or unwanted initially, it does not follow automatically that the child would remain unwanted or unloved. In general most parents become appropriately invested in the child as the pregnancy proceeds or after the child is born.) How did the parents adjust to the pregnancy? What was the mother's/father's predominant emotional state during pregnancy? Was the child born full term or premature? Was it a normal delivery? Were there any complications during labor, delivery, or postnatal period? Cesarean section, or one that required another type of assistance? What was the birth weight? Did the child reach the usual developmental milestones at expected times, or were they significantly delayed? Inquire specifically about when the child first rolled over, sat up, and, most important, started walking and talking. Inquire about the development of speech: when the child started saying the first words, phrases, and sentences; whether the child was talkative or quiet to any unusual degree. Inquire whether there was any lag or arrest in speech development. If so what remedial measures where undertaken, and what were the results? Ask about the appearance of smile, and how the child responded to the parents' affectionate behavior toward him or her. Inquire when the child attained bowel and bladder control. Inquire about the child's early temperament. Was this a child who was easy to interact with, or did the child have a difficult temperament? Was the child difficult to please, manage, and extremely demanding? Have such problems persisted or improved significantly? What were the child's sleep patterns during infancy, preschool years, and later? Was the child under-active, normally active, or hyperactive during infancy and later?

4. School and Social History

Inquire how the child adjusted to beginning school. Was there significant separation problem or school phobic behavior? Were there significant behavior or discipline problems in school? If yes, how were they dealt with? If there are significant academic problems, were they present since early elementary school years, or did they start manifesting only during adolescence. Are there indications of significant learning disabilities? If there are, which are the learning capacities affected? If there are learning disabilities, how has the problem been dealt with? Inquire about the child's attitude toward homework. Is it something that he can mostly manage independently or do the parents have to be involved in the process excessively? Inquire about the adolescent's expectations for himself or herself regarding academics and future career choices, how they compare to the parental expectations for him or her, and if there is a serious disparity between the two, how is the difference of opinion dealt with? Are the parents and child, normally concerned, unconcerned, or overly concerned and over anxious about tests, grades, etc.? Are studies over emphasized in the household to the point that the other developmental needs of the child are neglected?

Inquire if the child is interested in and involved with his or her peers in the community. Is this family appropriately socially involved or isolated? Do they feel reasonably comfortable in the world around them, or do they feel uncomfortable and out of place, and if so why? (Such inquiries are especially pertinent with the families of many immigrant and minority children.) An informal assessment should be made of the general social and interpersonal skills of the child and parents.

5. Parent's relationship to the child and parent's perception of the child's problems

Ascertain if there is genuine affection and concern for this child from parent's or guardians or if they appear to be only angry and hostile to the child. Do they have difficulty expressing affection toward the child? Is the interaction with the child mostly in the form of criticisms of his or her performance or shortcomings? How is the child disciplined? Is there a history of physical punishment or threats? (If there is, the parents should be advised in a supportive manner how important it is to refrain from such behavior and how destructive such actions are for the child and their mutual relationship. The clinician may have to initiate actions of informing the designated authorities if he or she suspects that a child is being abused or significantly neglected.) Determine if the child's relationship to the parents is based primarily on trust and affection or on fear and hostility. Ascertain if the parents favor one or more among their children. If they do, do they know why? Inquire as to what the parents think is happening to their child and what measures they think could be helpful. Make a determination as to whether they see the child's problems mainly as "bad behavior" needing disciplinary measures only; or being due to environmental stresses requiring environmental manipulations, or to be addressed by advice, counseling or other psychotherapeutic measures only; or one that needs treatment with medicines. Inquire whether they are open to suggestions that differ from how they feel the problem should be dealt with. (This area of inquiry is very important in formulating a treatment plan that may be acceptable to the parents.)

6. Family history of psychiatric problems and functioning of the family

This is arguably the most sensitive area in the interview with the parents. Inquire if any of the parents have a history of psychiatric illness, whether identified and treated as such or not. If there is, what were the manifestations, the course of the illness, and response to treatment? Also, inquire if any of the siblings, grandparents, uncles and aunts, and first cousins on maternal or paternal side has suffered from similar or related problems? Inquire about alcoholism or drug abuse among family members, including the personality functioning of any relative so affected. This inquiry is important because not only is there a tendency for alcoholism and other substance abuse to afflict several family members, but also many people suffering from affective illnesses, especially bipolar disorders, are often referred to by family members and others as having the problem of alcoholism or drug use only, with the manifestations of affective illness not recognized correctly, especially because of the complicating alcohol or substance abuse, or because of the families' reluctance to acknowledge or accept mental illness in one of their own.

In this context it is important to note that, just because a parent or family member is identified as suffering from a particular psychiatric illness or problem, it does not mean that the child's problems are manifestations of the same illness or problem. In fact often the child may be reacting to the stresses caused by illness in a parent or family member. However one psychiatric illness—bipolar disorder—in a parent, grand parent, or sibling, warrants that special attention should be given to determine if the child's serious behavioral or emotional problems are an early manifestation of this illness or its related vulnerabilities, considering the high penetrance of this genetic illness through generations and considering the fact that this illness is so much more common among children than most professionals consider it to be, especially in children who are exhibiting severe behavior problems (including hyperactivity) or depression. Inquiry on such matters should be conducted in a very supportive and sensitive manner, as it provokes and sets in motion emotional upheaval and concerns in the parents, but it is nevertheless an area that needs careful probing to complete a good evaluation. If the parents appear defensive and purposefully vague in their replies, do not persist with the inquiry to the point of breaching the rapport with them or making them very uncomfortable. With experience, sensitivity, and an appreciation of the importance of this area of inquiry, one is often able to elicit much valuable information and assess its relative importance in the child's problems. At times an opportunity to meet with grandparents or siblings will provide additional opportunity for data gathering in this area by observation or inquiry.

Inquire about the parent's own childhood, their families of origin, values their parents inculcated in them (and what values they inculcate in their children), their goals when growing up, their level of satisfaction or dissatisfaction with life, major reasons for unhappiness if any, parents' general philosophy of life, religious beliefs, how flexible or inflexible their belief systems are, etc., as appropriate to a particular situation or presenting problem. Assess how the parents get along with each other and how the child's problems impact on their relationship. Do they agree or disagree on how to deal with the child's problems? Are they blaming each other for the child's problems?

7. Medical and Neurological history

Inquire if the child has any medical problems, acute or chronic. If the child does have a significant medical problem, ascertain whether the psychiatric problems could be directly or indirectly related to it. Is there a history of hospitalizations of significance? Is there any history of prolonged anesthesia? Is there a history of seizure disorder? Make a determination as to how any medical/neurological problem may be impacting on the child biologically and/or psychologically. It is important to know of the medical status of the child, not only in arriving at a proper diagnosis, but also in deciding on the nature of treatment measures, especially pharmacotherapy which impacts on multiple systems.

Chapter IV

The Evaluation—Part II

Interviewing the child and Mental Status Examination

Ideally the child should be prepared for the interview in advance by the parents and /or referring person as to the nature of the visit. If properly done this will help minimize fear and negativism in the child. In general for the purpose of the evaluation, children can be categorized into four age or developmental groups: the preschool child, the early elementary school child, the middle school or junior high school age child, and the adolescent or high school age child. Some general points regarding interviewing children and adolescents are mentioned below.

The Use of play

Much has been written about the use of play, especially its symbolic significance in the assessment and treatment of children. There is no doubt that play acts as a medium that allows for better observation and evaluation of the young child's spontaneous activity and verbalizations, as well as provides inroads to their interests, preoccupations, and concerns. However, the overemphasis on play as a diagnostic and therapeutic tool, especially the overemphasis on symbolic interpretation of play along psychoanalytic lines, is of very little value in the psychiatric evaluation of children. This should in no way be construed as saying that play does not have a significant role in the evaluation and treatment of young children. It is useful to keep in mind a few points regarding the use of play in this context.

Play serves the purpose of diffusing tension and putting the child at ease so that anxiety-laden topics can be probed gently as opportunities arise. Spontaneous and structured play also provide additional means and in some children a better opportunity than in a face-to-face interview, to assess the activity level, cognitive, representational and symbolic capacity, capacity to concentrate, distractibility, impulsivity, and capacity to follow adult directions, among others. In addition in the preschool and early elementary school age child, concerns and conflicts that are difficult for them to articulate well in a face-to-face interview often emerge as themes during their play activity. Children provide glimpses of their habitual ways of dealing with the world around them during their play activities, and their spontaneous verbalizations during play give openings for the careful observer to further explore their concerns and conflicts.

If not properly used, play could become a hindrance in pursuing meaningful verbal interchange with the child and a form of avoidance in dealing with important issues in psychotherapy. It is the responsibility of the clinician to skillfully use the playtime so that, meaningful information may be obtained from the time spend and to justify the expenses incurred by parents or third parties. Too often clinicians introduce the child to play activities with little forethought as to the goals to be accomplished and how to accomplish them, leading to unproductive or chaotic sessions from which little is gained. It is not unusual to see young children coming to clinics week after week for play sessions, with little if any meaningful information or therapeutic benefit obtained, as the clinician is unsure of what is to be accomplished by the use of play.

Ideally the younger children are interviewed and observed in a room with at least a minimum amount of play materials that could be used for spontaneous and, when necessary, structured play. It is important to avoid having materials that could be used by an impulsive child in a dangerous or chaotic manner. A doll house with accompanying articles and doll figures, puppets representing family members, puzzles that can be put together without having to spend too much time, toy cars and trucks, simple two-person interactive board games, model building sets, sets of crayons, pencils, and a supply of papers for drawing and writing, are adequate for most evaluation purposes. A great deal of spontaneous play activity by the child could be observed even with minimal amounts of play materials provided, if the child's interest is channeled skillfully by the interviewer to materials that are likely to provide the most information in a given situation. Clinicians often overstock an excessive amount and variety of play materials. This is often unnecessary and even detracts rather than being helpful in conducting proper evaluation, with the child being distracted by the sheer amount and variety of objects around and often moving from one play material to other in a haphazard manner, revealing little information and making assessment of various aspects of the child's functioning difficult and open to question because of the distracting atmosphere.

Combining Play and Face-to-Face Interactions

All preschool and early elementary school age children should be given an opportunity to use play materials, at least to some extent, as part of the evaluation process. Much information can also be obtained by providing a paper and pencil and asking the school age child to use it for drawing, copying geometrical figures, and writing. All children should be encouraged to take part in direct verbal interchange that could be slowly guided towards the presenting problems and related issues without raising the discomfort level of the child too much. The preschool child and the early elementary school age child are best interviewed and observed through a combination of play and face-to-face interview and the upper elementary school age child and the adolescent mostly by direct interview, though paper and pencil tasks and activities are very relevant, if not essential, and helpful in these age groups also.

The Interview Process

In evaluating adults, usually the interviewer starts by asking what the presenting problem is. In the case of children, more often than not, this approach is to be avoided because others who have detected the need for an evaluation bring them, and the child may only have a vague idea why he is seeing the psychiatrist. Even though the older children may be aware of why they may be seeing the psychiatrist -albeit only vaguely in some cases-, often it is quite uncomfortable for them to talk about it, especially to strangers. Hence the early part of the evaluation should be spent in making the child feel at ease and in developing rapport.

This could be achieved with the younger child by either letting the child play, with the interviewer introducing a verbal interchange aimed at putting the child at ease and setting the tone for the interview, or by introducing and talking about neutral or pleasurable topics, such as what kind of things they like to do, life at home and school, their friends, any interesting and pleasant things that happened recently, their family, their plans and wishes for the future, hobbies, television shows they like, areas in which they may have had creditable achievement, etc. As the interview progresses and rapport is established, there may be opportunities to bring up and explore issues related to the presenting problem and related concerns and conflicts. It is important to avoid raising the discomfort level of the child beyond a reasonable and tolerable level when exploring these issues. It would be helpful to keep in mind that the clinician's role is not that of a policeman or judge, but rather of one who tries to understand the child's feelings, experiences and concerns, what may be making him or her act one way or another, and what could be done to improve the situation.

A great deal of information is often obtained from younger children if a playful quality is introduced into the interview, provided it is appropriate for the present mental state and circumstances of the child (In a child who is significantly or acutely distressed one would of course not use such a light-hearted approach). In the interview of children, a great deal depends on the "educated guess" the evaluator has about the child's problems and concerns. Rather than question the child, especially the younger child, directly about these possibilities, it is often more fruitful to pose the questions in a hypothetical or indirect manner. For example, if the interviewer suspects that the anxiety generated because of her mother's and other family members' response to the diagnosis of a possible cancerous illness in the mother may be underlying the recent problematic separation anxiety and school phobia in a six-year-old child, rather than ask "are you afraid your mother is going to die?" the interviewer may ask while the child is engaged in play with family doll figures, "Supposing there was this little girl and this mummy, and supposing the mummy was not feeling well and had to go to the hospital for check-ups and operations and things like that, what will happen to the little girl, do you think? You think she'll be sad? Scared? What kind of worries do you think she'll have? Who can help her with her worries do you think? Who do you think can help her and look after her when the mummy is in the hospital? When is she going to be most worried and scared you think? What can she do not to be so scared? Is there someone who can help her not to be too scared and upset?" etc. Another technique is to acknowledge that the interviewer has seen many children in similar circumstances as he or she is and ask, if by chance, he or she may be experiencing particular emotions or concerns that have been common in those children. This may help children elaborate on their inner feelings and concerns.

Identifying some serious but not uncommon psychiatric disorders or problems in children requires a great deal of experience on the part of the clinician by gaining relevant experience in dealing with severely troubled children under supervisors who are well experienced with such problems. For example clinicians often are at a loss as to how to approach a child who may be experiencing suicidal thoughts or auditory hallucinations. Of a child who is suspected to be experiencing suicidal thoughts, one may inquire "When you feel so bad or upset sometimes, do you feel like it is better not to be living? Do you get thoughts in your mind that you should hurt yourself?" If the child acknowledges such thoughts or impulses, go on to gently explore how strong the thought or impulse may be. Explore in a calm and supportive manner with questions such as: "Those thoughts, do they bother you a lot? Do they keep coming back again and again? How do they make you feel? Can you ignore them? etc. If the child acknowledges intense suicidal thoughts, urges, or death wishes, gently ask if he experiences these as thoughts, or as his mind or someone else telling him to end his life or that he is better off dead. If the child acknowledges a voice, ask whose voice it sounds like. Any child who experiences strong suicidal thoughts or urges, of course has to be further queried about any methods he or she feels like employing to end his or her life. Often children who are predisposed to experiencing intense emotionality when upset report, on probing, a voice in their "brain" or "head" telling them to stab, kill themselves, etc.

Also, susceptible children who frequently go into uncontrollable rages, fighting and generally out of control behavior which often give the appearance of "bizarreness" to their behavior and actions when they are in such states, acknowledge on careful probing an urging or voice in their "head" or "brain"—that of their own mind which they identify as such, or the voice of another known or unknown person—urging them to "fight", "beat up" others, "run around", "be bad", "don't listen" etc. Children often report such phenomena as occurring when they feel provoked by or angry with someone. These tendencies and phenomena go undetected in many severely troubled children because of the interviewer's inability to suspect the presence of such phenomena and to skillfully probe to clarify the nature of such experiences. For clinicians and others, such thoughts and experiences in a child are naturally unsettling, further interfering with their capacity to elicit such information and to arrive upon proper conclusions unless they have had a strong interest and proper training to address such issues. A good deal of experience in dealing with severely ill and troubled children and an in depth understanding of severe psychopathology in children are required to effectively evaluate and understand such problems.

There are several general areas to be covered during the interview and mental status examination with the child. The following guidelines could be helpful, if used in a flexible manner, to conduct a reasonable and generally adequate evaluation in most clinical situations. It is important that the interviewer should obtain an understanding of what the child thinks of the reported presenting problem and related issues. As mentioned before, this does not mean the interview should start with exploration of the presenting problem. By the time the interview and observation sessions are concluded, one should have as good an understanding as possible as to how the child experiences and understands the problems.

Generally within a few minutes of meeting a youngster, the interviewer can make a determination if he or she will be able to conduct a reasonably free-flowing interview, or whether the special problems posed by the youngster, usually due to lack of cooperation or because of the nature of the disturbance the child is experiencing (for example: psychosis, mania, severe depression, or major developmental problems), calls for deviating from the usual format, needing great deal of innovation depending on the circumstances. Sufficient information can be gleaned from most children, even if they are not very cooperative, to arrive at a tentative formulation, diagnostic understanding, and preliminary treatment plan.

Interviewing the Preschool child

Most preschool children seen in clinical situations are either quite spontaneous or the opposite: inhibited, anxious and clinging excessively to their parents. With most children one can start the interview by helping the child to feel comfortable with the interviewer and the environment by engaging the child in conversation, starting with their name, how old they are, names of their siblings, friends, things they enjoy, etc. From this initial getting acquainted phase, one could proceed with introducing the child to the toys available and helping the child engage in play activities, while at the same time weaving in topics that may be related to the presenting problem, for which opportunities almost always arise during their play.

For example, in a four or five-year-old, suspected to be exhibiting increased emotionality, oppositional tendencies, temper tantrums, excessive aggression, and related problems precipitated by recent parental divorce, one would introduce the child to the doll house, observe the play, and simultaneously introduce questions about the parental doll figures, their relationship, and what is happening to the child or children who make up the family. Often this will give glimpses of the child's inner life and concerns related to the parental situation. The child could later be engaged in more face-to-face interactions aimed at assessing among other things his cognitive level, ability to remain seated, speech and language capacities, capacity to relate, and capacity to engage in meaningful verbal interchange about his or her problems and related issues. It is appropriate to introduce crayon or pencil and paper tasks appropriate for their age for children over three years of age. Just asking a child to copy a circle or square and to print his or her name and observing the child's response can reveal a wealth of information. These tasks help identify among others, the child's receptive language capacity, ability to be cooperative, oppositional and impulsive tendencies, eye-hand and fine motor coordination, attention and concentration, and ability to follow directions. One could also glean information on the inner life, desires, and longings of children as young as four by asking them to state their three magic wishes. A 60minute session with a child of this age group, following a good information gathering session with the parents, will usually yield sufficient preliminary data to reach tentative conclusions about the child and her problems.

A frightened, resistant, and clinging preschooler, on the other hand, would require a different approach. Once a child is found to be clinging to the parents excessively in a frightened or resistant and anxious manner, an attempt should be made to allay the child's anxieties about the evaluation process by explaining what the process would be like, how benign or even enjoyable it could be with an opportunity to explore the toys, play, etc., and that there won't be any painful procedures such as injections (many preschool and young children equate visiting the doctor or clinics with painful procedures such as injections and blood drawing). If the child continues to be frightened and resistant there is no good reason to persist with the attempt to see the child alone during the preliminary visit. Obviously for such a child the ability to trust others in an age appropriate manner and to separate from the parents to a reasonable degree would be a task to accomplish as part of the treatment process.

A child who cannot separate from the parents even for a play session will have to be observed and evaluated in the presence of the parents. I would tell such a child that it is not absolutely necessary to be in the office and play area without the parents and that the parents could be with him or her, and that later perhaps he or she will feel comfortable to let the parents go out and be in the waiting area. Many children who initially have difficulty separating from the parents feel comfortable enough to let the parents leave the office and be in the waiting area once they feel at ease with the evaluator and the setting during the play session. For a small minority of children, separation from parents even for brief periods is an impossible task, which will have to be addressed in treatment gradually. Sometimes it may be the main presenting problem itself.

Often trainees are distressed when having to deal with the children who refuse to enter the office or separate from the parents even for brief periods and start crying or throwing temper tantrums, not knowing how to proceed with the evaluation and experiencing it as a sign of incompetence on their part. Such children often evoke negative feelings in the evaluator. Beginners in the field often spend an inordinate amount of time and effort to accomplish the separation in the initial session itself. There is little need for this. Once a determination is made from initial interactions that the child has such severe difficulty, one should change the approach and try to gain as much information as possible by not insisting that the child separate from the parents for the evaluation, but observing the child in the presence of the parents while trying to console him or her. With an extremely frightened or resistant child who refuses to enter the office even with the parents, one could continue the supportive, reassuring engagement in the waiting area itself, including bringing the toys and other materials there and encouraging the child to explore them. Whatever the child would or would not do in such a situation provides significant information about the child's capacities and deficiencies. Many such children would feel comfortable being in the office later on or during the next visit. Even if they do not, that information itself is highly revealing of the child and his problems and in selecting the therapeutic approach to be recommended. Obviously the more frightened and resistant the child is the more time will have to be apportioned to complete the evaluation by scheduling extra visits as needed. Trainees should take comfort in the thought that, in general a child who is difficult to evaluate for them would prove to be difficult for even experienced clinicians.

The question often comes up as to why a four or five-year-old needs to be seen alone as part of the evaluation process (a child younger than three is best evaluated in the presence of the parents in most circumstances). There are several reasons why it is important to observe and interact with a child with and without the parents or guardian present. The presence of the parents or guardian would influence the behavior and utterances of the child one way or another. The presence of the parents would affect to varying degrees the spontaneous interaction and conversation between the child and the evaluator, generally playing an inhibitory role in the interaction and verbal exchange, depending on the experience of the therapist and how comfortable the child may feel revealing certain concerns in front of one parent, the other, or the guardian, and how controlling, interfering, or cooperative the parent is, etc. This is especially so in situations where there are parent-child conflicts or conflicts between the parents that affect the child. Foster children often feel uncomfortable talking about concerns about their foster status, or their thoughts and concerns about their biological parents and related issues in front of the foster parents. It is very difficult to ask probing questions even in a careful, sensitive, and gentle manner with children suspected to be experiencing certain phenomena such as psychosis, including hallucinations, or suicidal urges, in the presence of parents. These are but a few examples of why an evaluation is more likely to be complete if the child is seen both with and without the parents or guardian present. In the case of older children and adolescents, if they are not seen with and without the parents being present, the evaluation will have to be considered incomplete to that extent.

Interviewing The Elementary School Child

The younger of the elementary school age children are evaluated with a format resembling that of the older preschoolers described previously. As the children's age and developmental level advance there is more emphasis and time spent on attempts at face-to-face verbal interchange and less time and emphasis on play in general. With a preschool child, the usual technique is to introduce the child to play activities early in the session and come back to more direct verbal explorations later. With an elementary school age child, especially among the older group of these children, it is best to spend significant time in direct verbal interchange, to assess the child's functioning and capacity in general, and to explore concerns and questions related to the presenting problem. Again these formats should not be rigid. One generally follows the child's lead, assessing what comes easily and spontaneously to them and then trying to channel the session skillfully to obtain the maximum amount of information possible while keeping the child interested and not unduly anxious in the process. Some of the very young among the elementary school age children would have little difficulty entering into a very productive verbal interchange soon after meeting the clinician, whereas some older children would give one word vague answers at best during the initial phase of the encounter, necessitating the interviewer to introduce paper and pencil tasks, including drawing and an invitation to explore the toys and other play materials early in the session.

Many elementary school age children are seen for problems related to hyperactivity, impulsivity, and aggression. Many such children would have difficulty sitting down for a face-to-face verbal interchange for any significant length of time. Such children would require a very flexible approach, combining activities including play, face-to-face verbal interchange, and short periods of paper and pencil activities. Many such children would just want to play, and an often useful technique in evaluating such children is to say that the clinician would like to talk to them and have them do a few paper and pencil tasks, after which they could engage in play for a sufficient amount of time. Many children are able to adhere reasonably to such formats, though their attention and interest in the task may have to be refocused time and again. How well they are able to adhere to such formats reveals a great deal about their capacities and functioning. Once a child is found to be very hyperactive and impulsive, the clinician will have to take efforts to structure the session more, otherwise all one would understand will be just how hyperactive and impulsive the child can be.

Interviewing The Preadolescent and Adolescent/Teen-ager

Generally the evaluation could proceed primarily with verbal interchange and paper and pencil tasks in the preadolescent and adolescent, provided the youngster is reasonably cooperative. After a brief introductory period when the evaluator meets the youngster with his parents, makes a preliminary assessment of the situation, and apprises the child and parents of the general format of the evaluation, one could proceed to meet with the parents alone to gather background information, including the presenting concerns and problems, followed by interview with the youngster.

Compared to a younger child, with whom indirect probing and play are utilized to a greater degree, with an older child or adolescent, after an initial phase utilized to put the youngster at ease with questions aimed at non-problematic areas and supportive statements, one proceeds to exploring issues that are aimed at problem areas in an empathic and supportive manner. In most youngsters of these age groups, paper and pencil tasks, including obtaining a writing sample and doing simple arithmetic operations (especially in youngsters suspected to have cognitive deficiencies), would be very helpful. Special skills are called for when youngsters of these age groups are very angry and resistant to being interviewed. Most of these youngsters have some understanding as to why they are brought to see the evaluator though they may not always overtly acknowledge it, may have some misunderstanding about it, or may disagree as to what they perceive the problem to be compared to what the parents or school authorities may perceive the problem to be. Depending on the level of uncooperativeness or hostility evident, the approach of the interview will have to be modified, often in an innovative manner appropriate to the situation.

In general the evaluator has to maintain objectivity in the presence of uncooperative or provocative behavior and statements on the part of these youngsters. It helps to remind oneself that what appears to be willful behavior on the part of these youngsters is more often than not a manifestation of their psychiatric illness and may not be within their easy control, as it may often appear to be. It is often helpful to inform the youngster that the clinician is aware of the general nature of the problem as others perceive it, and is interested in knowing how the youngster himself or herself perceives it, so that whatever helpful measures possible could be suggested to ameliorate the situation. Such efforts, when presented in a genuine, concerned, and empathic manner, will often help the youngster cooperate at least to a degree with the evaluation.

Trainees often feel unhappy and distressed that these difficult to evaluate youngsters do not talk or do not give enough information to accomplish a reasonable evaluation. As in the case of the younger resistant or frightened child, it is helpful to keep in mind that one gathers valuable information from the resistant and angry behavior itself, as it sheds light on the very nature and intensity of the youngster's difficulties and the difficulties that will have to be surmounted in treatment.

Adolescents often protest that they are not "crazy" and don't need to see a "stupid shrink." Behind these protests lie the fear and stigma of mental illness and the fear of being misunderstood and mistreated (legitimate concerns for anyone in their predicament.) A sympathetic explanation that the psychiatrist's interest is in hearing their side of the story, making them feel better, and reducing the misunderstanding or conflict between them and others will often help to reduce such resistance. Pointing out an often evident fact that they are sensitive people whose feelings are easily hurt, and that when upset or angry they may have difficulty controlling what they say and how they act (which is almost always true of such resistant and angry youngsters) in an appropriate and relevant manner will also help many of these youngsters become more cooperative, as they feel the psychiatrist has experience dealing with the kind of difficulties they may be experiencing. The clinician who is confident of his or her commitment in being of help to such youngsters can reduce the resistance of most and help them open up, at least to some degree. Not reacting to the youngster's resistant and provocative behavior with anger, rejection and an uncaring attitude (which such behavior often provoke in the clinician) is crucial in having any success at all with such youngsters.

The youngsters who are totally resistant or explosive and aggressive inspite of the clinician's earnest, supportive approach are often too troubled to be helped in the out-patient setting in the present circumstances and may need other interventions if the presenting problems are serious enough, such as admission to an in-patient unit or residential setting. When dealing with such difficult and troubled youngsters, the clinician need not feel inadequate, as dealing with such youngsters is among the most difficult and emotionally stressful situations one could face in the whole field of medicine and psychiatry.

Dealing with Special populations such as The Mentally Retarded and Autistic Children

The evaluation approach has to be modified when one is dealing with children who are cognitively limited or suffer from related developmental disorders such as autism. Even though the primary focus in evaluating such children is to determine the level of their functioning, strengths, deficiencies etc.,—including the often accompanying and difficult to manage or troublesome hyperactivity, impulsivity, self and other directed aggression, and related behavior problems—it is wise to keep in mind that even the most obviously retarded or autistic youngster is equally prone to other mental illnesses that are common in children of normal intelligence.

It is wise to pay special attention to the office or venue in which such children would be evaluated, especially if the evaluation is for severe behavior and impulse control problems. Many such children are extremely impulsive—generally more so than children of normal intelligence. Because many have limited language capacity if any, verbal interventions are not very effective in curbing their impulsivity. They tend to become over-stimulated and highly impulsive if they are brought into an office with a plethora of toys and other objects, especially such objects on the clinician's table. Many such children impulsively lunge, grab, mishandle and damage objects in the office, especially equipment on the office table. A great deal of the clinician's and parents' time and energy would be wasted in trying to prevent them from engaging in such activities. Hence it is wise that arrangements be made to evaluate such children in an office or space that has only the essential materials required for such an evaluation, and where other objects are kept to an essential minimum and out of reach from the children.

One of the most frequent problems overlooked in such youngsters, even by experienced clinicians is bipolar disorder, which presents primarily as behavioral worsening only in these youngsters as they are often non verbal, and hence even the most common feature of classical mania—over-talkativeness and pressured speech—are not present to arouse suspicion in the clinician as to the presence of this illness. Unless the clinician maintains a healthy index of suspicion to rule out the presence of this and related disorders and makes necessary inquiry regarding the possible waxing and waning nature of the child's problems, manifestations of changes in energy level and physical activity, and sleep problems, and also probes the family history for incidences of such illnesses or problems highly suggestive of the occurrence of such illnesses, one could miss identifying even a full blown manic or depressive, episode in such youngsters. It is not unusual to see such youngsters go through highly troublesome manic episodes that endanger their safety and that of others time and again, with clinicians failing to recognize the illness even though the child may have been seen even in emergency room visits by several clinicians.

There is a general lack of awareness that a youngster exhibiting mental retardation, or autistic and related disorders has as equal a chance as a child who is not so affected to suffer from bipolar and related disorders. Identifying such serious mental illnesses in these special populations of youngsters is one of the most helpful skills a child psychiatrist can develop through proper training under good supervision from clinicians experienced in such matters. It is the lack of such skills on the part of the clinicians that often makes these youngsters go from one clinic to another and visit emergency rooms in crises repeatedly with little relief coming their way. Often clinicians attribute all behavioral problems in such youngsters as a manifestation of mental retardation or autism only, or to Attention Deficit Hyperactive Disorder (ADHD) and deny them badly needed in-patient admission and interventions when they go through such manic episodes, compounding the distress of the children, their families, and other caregivers and subjecting everyone involved to unnecessary physical and emotional trauma.

Since many mentally retarded and autistic youngsters have very little verbal capacity, if any, more time has to be spent gathering a detailed history of their behavior problems from parents and other caregivers, including school personnel, and in observing their behavior, often through several sessions. A final diagnosis or ruling out of an illness, such as bipolar disorder, in some of these children is only possible after seeing them over a period of time in follow up visits as the problem tends to improve at least partially and worsen periodically, revealing its nature. This wait is worth the trouble, as it will prevent the child from being misunderstood, misdiagnosed and mistreated if such episodes recur in the future (as they most often do.)

Becoming competent in the psychiatric evaluation of developmentally disordered and mentally retarded children is a special skill that requires continued work with such populations under the guidance of supervisors who are truly experienced in the evaluation and treatment of such children and their psychiatric problems. This usually will require training and working in a venue in which large numbers of such children are evaluated and treated, for a period extending beyond the formal training period in child psychiatry.

The Flow of the Interview

The purpose of the interview is to gain as much relevant information about the child and his or her problems and also to make mental status observations, leading to a comprehensive understanding of the child, including arriving upon the most likely diagnoses so that appropriate treatment measures can be implemented if indicated. A good evaluator follows the child's lead yet keeps the verbalizations and interactions focused on obtaining maximum relevant information within the allotted period. Toward the latter part of the session, special attempts are made to focus the child's attention on important issues that have not been touched upon during the unstructured early part of the session. (Often out of necessity to make a child feel comfortable and observe the spontaneous behavior and verbalizations, the early part of the interview is kept relatively unstructured and free flowing.) The interview and observations form the basis for forming a mental status of the child, which is important in arriving at appropriate diagnoses and in forming a describable mental picture of the child as he or she presents during the evaluation period.

Mental Status Examination

The mental status is the synthesis and interpretation of observational data regarding the mental functioning and behavior of the child presented in a concise format. Throughout the evaluation session the clinician should be observing and making determinations regarding the various aspects of the child's mental status. Mental status examination is an integral part of the whole evaluation and not separate from it. The following general areas should be covered as part of the mental status examination of children.

General Appearance and Behavior

Observe the appearance of the child. Does he look his or her age, appear physically healthy, or unwell? Are there obvious dysmorphic features? Observe the attire and grooming. What about the general demeanor of the child and his relatedness? Is he reasonably cooperative, or very resistant and hostile, or unusually fearful or shy? Are there any striking separation problems from the parents? Much more than what one would expect from a child of his or her age?

Note that most children, especially the older children whose overall functioning is in the average range, come across as some what inhibited during the initial phases of the interview. Lack of such normal social inhibition, in the form of intrusive behavior, impulsivity, and indiscriminate over-talkativeness, often gives the first clue as to the likely general nature of the problem. Also signs of significant developmental delays or disorders are often evident within a short time of meeting the child from his or her appearance, general behavior, speech, and manner of relating. Note the activity level of the child. Is he or she normally active, under active, or over active? What about impulsivity? Note also that many hyperactive and impulsive children will not exhibit such features in a significant manner when seen in a one-on-one interview with an adult authority figure who is a stranger to them. Observations during spontaneous play and while in the waiting area, and when with other children or siblings, and in less restrictive settings would be more revealing about this aspect of the child's functioning. This is one of the reasons why teacher reports are extremely useful in identifying such problems, especially when there is great disparity between what the parents report and what the clinician observes in the initial interview.

In this context one should also keep in mind that what one observes in a clinical interview setting is at best only an approximation of the child's behavior in his "natural environment." Just because a child appears not to be very hyperactive, impulsive, or aggressive when seen in the office, one should not disbelieve the parents' or teacher's report that the child has such problems. However, if one has not been able to verify such behavior by direct observation one should suspend a final opinion on the matter until further observations—if necessary by home or school visit—and information from other sources become available.

Observe also whether the child appears well coordinated in his or her movements or actions or if there are indications of a poorly coordinated neuromuscular system. Such observations give indication as to whether a more detailed neurological evaluation would be necessary. It is a good practice to observe the gait of all children, especially those in whom developmental problems are suspected or present. Unsteady or unusual gait is a strong indicator of neurodevelopmental and related problems

Intelligence

Make a general estimate of the child's cognitive functioning from the manner in which the child conducts himself or herself, the verbal capacity (or non-verbal communication capacity in a nonverbal child), the general knowledge the child exhibits, the social awareness or lack of it exhibited, the child's capacity for self-care, the academic capacities the child possesses in the case of the school age child, and related capacities. If there are obvious concerns about the child's cognitive capacities, the child will have to be referred for psychological testing to ascertain cognitive and related capacities if it has not been done already.

Speech and Language

Observe the speech and language capacities of the child. Are there significant problems in articulation, fluency of speech, the level of vocabulary, and receptive and expressive language capacities? Is there evidence of distorted or deviant language use indicative of a formal thought disorder? Is the child echolalic beyond what is expected for his or her age? (This most often points to a significant developmental disorder.) Note also if the child exhibits particular preoccupations or mixing of fantasy and reality beyond what is expected for his age. Make a special observation whether the child appears, extremely over-talkative, or his expressions show a lack of normal inhibitions. Though over-talkativeness could be a normal variation up to a degree, extreme over-talkativeness—especially without appropriate social inhibitions—is often a strong indicator of a possible mood disorder, such as bipolar disorder, when accompanied by other related pathological phenomena. At the opposite end of this are children who appear selectively mute, again pointing to possible serious pathological conditions.

Mood and affect

Observe what the general mood of the child is and the affective range and variations observed. Is the child depressed? Irritable? If so, assess the intensity of these. Observe for Additional features of depression and other mood disorders, such as lability of mood, pathological excitability, or euphoria.

In younger children, since separating from parents often would be a major problem in the interview setting, with the attendant anxiety, tearfulness etc. the child would exhibit, determining what the prevailing mood of the child would be in a more natural environment such as the home or even school may be difficult. Observe the level of anxiety and fear the child exhibits when separating and also whether the anxiety and distress diminishes appropriately with reassurance and encouragement from the parents and clinician. If it becomes very difficult for the child to separate from the parents, do not insist on it to an unreasonable degree. Many younger children, especially of preschool age, as mentioned before, may have to be interviewed in the parent's presence because of separation problems. Whenever possible, however, an attempt should be made to see the child with and without the parent or parents present to obtain optimal information and observational data. The evaluator has to develop skills as to how to conduct the interview of the child with and without the parents present.

Thought Processes

Determine if the thought processes are properly connected and goal oriented. (Often considerable experience is needed to make this determination in younger children who normally talk in a somewhat disjointed manner and in incomplete sentences and phrases.) Is there evidence for a formal thought disorder? (Note, one should not mistake expressive language disorder such as one sees in developmentally disordered children for formal thought disorder, which is a rare phenomenon in children.) Does the child show pressured speech, with sudden and frequent shifting from topic to topic? Does the child's thinking appear difficult to follow because of intermixing of fantasy or delusions and reality? (It will often require considerable experience and repeated observations to make such determinations in younger children.)

It is better to reserve judgment when one is uncertain on such matters, rather than hastily conclude that a child is experiencing psychotic phenomena or cannot distinguish fantasy and reality.

Fantasy life and Dreams

Try to ascertain what types of activities interest the child or preoccupy him or her. What does he or she want to be when they grow up? In older children and adolescents, what are the plans or methods to accomplish it? Asking the child what he or she would choose given three magic wishes is a time-honored and useful avenue to gain inroads to the wishes, fantasies, and preoccupations of children, without directly pressing them to reveal their inner desires, which many children fail to respond to in a useful manner. In response to such an inquiry, most children who are not significantly distressed about one thing or another will wish for a combination of material things that children in their particular culture value, at times along with a wish to be famous and rich, often combined with success in studies or their future career (especially with older children and adolescents), etc. Many children frequently wish for good things to happen for their parents and other family members or wish that their parents would never die and would live forever. Children who have particular preoccupations or worries often give glimpses of their concerns when answering this question. The very manner in which children approach this question itself may be highly revealing. Children who are depressed or highly distressed about one thing or another often have difficulty even coming up with three wishes. Some children who are very unhappy because of separation from or loss of a parent state just one wish: for the parent who died to be alive again.

Inquiring about any dreams of a repetitive nature or theme could also be revealing of the concerns, wishes, and fears of children.

Play

Observe the interest children show in play and play materials. Note how organized or impulsive and chaotic they may be in their approach to play and play materials. Pay attention to their spontaneous verbalizations during play. Note especially the appropriate or inappropriate use of play materials, including their capacity to use toys and play objects in a representative or symbolic manner. This is especially important in the evaluation of children who are cognitively impaired or suspected to be suffering from a pervasive developmental disorder such as autistic disorder, many of whom lack such capacity. Involvement in a simple two person board game that may have a competitive aspect to it helps to demonstrate a child's capacity to take part in meaningful interaction with another, to remain focused and goal directed, to tolerate frustration, and his or her cognitive skills and reaction to success or failure, among others. One has to be careful not to spend too much time exclusively in play during the evaluation, however, as this will limit the information one can obtain. Some children have difficulty disengaging from play once they are introduced to it and would require the skilled guidance of the clinician to make the session an appropriately comprehensive one including play and direct verbal interchange in reasonable proportion.

Special Symptoms

Inquire and observe for symptoms or phenomena such as obsessions, compulsions, phobias, hallucinations or delusions, or anything that stands out as unusual about the child's utterances or behavior. If one is unsure of what a particular behavior or utterance that appears unusual means, gently ask the child if he can explain that behavior or utterance.

Child's awareness of his or her problems

Make a determination as to whether the child has a general awareness as to the nature of his or her problems. Does he believe that he has a problem that requires help from those who deal with such problems? or does he think that he has no problems and that the parents and others are exaggerating or making false statements? Does he think that he is merely responding to the problems actually caused by others or that they are the people who really need help in improving their behavior or attitude, which causes his or her reactions? Determine if the child appears amenable to suggested interventions when the nature of the problem and the possible interventions that could be helpful are explained to him or her.

To cover all the areas mentioned above will obviously take a considerable amount of time, effort, and cooperation from the child. Not all areas, however, need to be covered in detail with all children. Clinicians should use their learned intuition and experience to decide which areas should be concentrated upon in detail with a particular child, depending on the nature of the presenting problems and the information obtained as the interview progresses.

Medical/Neurological Examination and Laboratory Studies

Psychiatric examination of the child is never complete without a good medical/ neurological examination. Whether the evaluating clinicians themselves should do the screening medical evaluation depends on the individual situation and the comfort level of the clinician in undertaking such tasks. The important point is that the evaluating psychiatrist should feel comfortable that he is well aware of the medical/neurological status of the child, whether he himself does the examination or whether another colleague or the child's own pediatrician conducts the examination. In most children who are under regular follow-up care from their pediatrician, a recent report from the doctor should provide most of the information that is necessary, to be supplemented by additional consultations, laboratory, or imaging studies, as the psychiatrist may consider relevant. Children in whom neurological or contributory medical problems are suspected should of course be referred to the relevant specialists for additional studies.

Evaluation and Synthesis of All Available Data, Diagnoses and Formulation

Once the interview and examinations are completed, the clinician should gather and review all the information obtained, including any school reports, psychological test reports, medical consultation reports, and laboratory reports that may be available. This should result in the clinician having a good understanding of the child and his problems in the bio-psycho-social sense, which should lead to a comprehensive formulation of the total situation and diagnoses using the standard, accepted nomenclature.

The formulation or case formulation is essentially a summary statement of the clinician's understanding of the child and his problems: how the child came to be how he or she is, what the problems are, and how they came to be. Consideration is given to all the factors: genetic-constitutional, family, environmental, and intra-psychic. Not only the deficiencies but also the strengths of the child should be mentioned, because often it is on the strengths that one is able to build a recovery and habilitation or rehabilitation. Each factor is weighed according to the major or minor role it plays in the production and maintenance of the problem or symptoms. As more information becomes available in the future, the formulation may have to be modified as appropriate.

Making formal diagnoses according to internationally accepted nomenclature and criteria is important, keeping in mind, however, the limitations involved. Diagnoses in child psychiatry are even more fluid and uncertain than in adult psychiatry, where also it remains mostly at an empirical, uncertain state. However, without formally diagnosing the problem it is difficult to formulate an appropriate treatment plan and communicate effectively with other professionals involved as to the general nature of the problem. For example it is important to know where the child's problems anchor: whether one is seeing most likely a transient reaction to a stressor in an otherwise healthy child, or whether the problem most likely is the manifestation of a more genetic/constitutionally based mental illness that is likely to run a more protracted course, or if the problem is primarily due to faulty brain structure or development. As further examples, it is important to know whether the child is most likely suffering from attention deficit hyperactivity disorder, bipolar disorder, a pervasive developmental disorder, or a conduct disorder because of the substantially different ways in which these problems have to be addressed and the varying onus of responsibility to be placed on the child and/or his parents in the remediation of his or her problems. In addition progress in the field depends on clinicians making as accurate a diagnosis as possible and matching it with treatment measures, to ascertain what works and what does not, and to understand how much of what types of problems exist in the community so that scarce research and financial resources can be allocated to the most pressing problems and in the most useful manner.

Informing the Parents and Child as to the Nature of the problem and what could Be Done About it

Once the clinician has come to a preliminary conclusion as to the nature of the child's problems, she (and if a team is involved in the evaluation preferably they also) should meet with the parents and, in lay terms explain to them in a supportive manner what the understandings are about the child and his problems and what measures could be helpful.

Depending on the age and the capacity of the child to understand helpful information, the nature of his or her problem, and measures that are suggested to bring about improvement this should also be explained in a comforting and supportive manner to the child in language that children of his or her developmental level can understand. If any information that is of very little therapeutic value and that could cause undue distress for the people concerned has surfaced during the evaluation, it should not be divulged in most circumstances. The clinicians' should use their good judgment in such unusual situations, keeping in mind that the first and foremost duty is to do no harm. The parents and child should be given an opportunity to ask any questions they may have about the feedback given to them and the measures suggested.

CHAPTER V

The Child Psychiatric Evaluation Report

The evaluation should result in a well-written Child Psychiatric Evaluation Report, documenting the problems, findings, and recommendations. It should contain the following elements:

Identifying Data

Date of Evaluation

Presenting problems (according to parents, other concerned adults, and the child, separately)

History of presenting problems and past history

History of any past treatment and response to treatment(s)

Developmental history

School and social history

Functioning of the family and relevant history of parents

Family psychiatric history

Medical/neurological history and significant findings

A brief description of the interview

(Give a brief narration of what transpired during the interview. This should include a brief description of the child and general behavior, pertinent observations from the child's play, and quotes from the child that may be highly revealing of the child and his problems and that would give the reader a vivid picture of the child, especially the type of information that cannot be conveyed fully in the mental status section.)

Mental Status

General description of child—appearance, general behavior, activity level, gait, gross and fine motor coordination, impulsivity, cooperativeness, relatedness, awareness of the surroundings, any unusual features etc.

Cognitive functioning—an estimate of the intelligence level and general knowledge of the child

Speech and language capacities—this should include how clear and well articulated the child's speech is, the receptive and expressive capacities, the volume and quantity of speech, any specific and significant features such as pressured speech, mutism etc.

Mood and affect—the prevailing mood of the child and the range and appropriateness of affect

Suicidal, homicidal, or assaultive tendencies

Thought processes/ preoccupations—presence or absence of formal thought disorder and related phenomena, any particular preoccupations evident etc.

Abnormal perceptual phenomena and special symptoms—the occurrence of any hallucinations, delusions, obsessions, compulsions, phobias, significant tics, motor abnormalities, etc, should be described here

Insight: child's awareness and understanding of his/her problems

Judgment: Child's capacity to act in a reasonable and age appropriate manner, especially when facing situations that call for thoughtful consideration of choices available

Formulation

This is a short paragraph as to the nature of the problem, contributing factors, and dynamic issues without being too speculative, theoretical, or abstract. When writing a formulation, make all attempts to make sure it would have practical relevance. Often clinicians write the formulation as if it is a theoretical exercise rife with jargon and outmoded ideas borrowed from speculative theories, which would have little relevance to the child's predicament or treatment. Another common error is to look for some far-fetched explanation for the child's problems, often simplistic in nature, and generally attributing all of the child's problems to some perceived minor defect in one parent or another or to a minor event in the past that is considered to have been so traumatic as to have caused a persistent, often severe psychiatric illness or disturbed behavior. Considering the fact that many of the problems seen in children are a result of a combination of factors biological, psychological, and social interacting to produce the given problem, it is wise to ascertain how much of what may be contributory in each case. In some cases the biological vulnerability may be the crucial factor, in another the extreme social stresses, in some severe parental neglect or abuse etc. It often takes great deal of honesty to oneself and experience, to produce formulations that are balanced, relevant, and provide the best understanding of the problem using the best of knowledge available about childhood psychopathology at that given time.

Diagnoses—as per accepted terminology in use

Recommendations—including treatment and any additional studies and other appropriate helpful measures

Chapter VI

Test Yourself

The following questions are intended to help the trainee think critically regarding issues that are relevant to psychiatric evaluations of children. Many of the topics dealt with in the questions have been discussed in one context or another in this book. The questions are followed by possible answers in multiple-choice format. Select the best answer, and write it down in the space for your answer. Think about your reasons for selecting the particular choice. Author's choice for the correct answer, and why the author thinks it is the best choice are given in the following page. The answers, and rationale for the particular choice being the correct answer are based on the author's experience and opinion only.

1. Child psychiatric evaluations of most children seen in clinics today, primarily depend on:
   a. Psychological testing
   b. Brain imaging and laboratory tests
   c. Psychoanalytic theory
   d. Interviewing the child and parents

   Your answer is:

Author's answer is (d): interviewing the child and parents. Psychological tests are helpful in determining the cognitive capacity of the child and related issues. They may be helpful in gaining insights into the child's habitual manner of dealing with the world around him or her, and the concerns and conflicts the child may be experiencing. Brain imaging and laboratory tests are presently only of limited clinical use in understanding the psychiatric problems of most children seen in evaluation. They are mostly research tools today. It is hoped that, in the future they will play a more important role, with advances in technology, as they become more effective in understanding mental phenomena and emotional states. Psychoanalytic theory provides very limited assistance in understanding, and dealing with the problems of most children seen today. At present, interviewing the child and parents is the most important and informative aspect of evaluation of children.

2. Psychiatric evaluation of children differs from that of adults, because:
   a. The need for evaluation is most often determined by someone other than the child
   b. The evaluation very often needs input from the school

c. Play is often a significant part of the evaluation

d. Interview and observation of the parents are very important

e. All of the above

Your answer is:

Author's choice is: (e), "All of the above". Most adults present themselves for evaluation because of one concern or another they may have, about themselves. In contrast most children are brought in for evaluation, because of concerns of parents', or school authorities about them. In evaluating an adult, it is the exception rather than the norm, that input from family members, his or her place of work etc. are solicited. In contrast, with children, input from parents is essential, and information from school is often necessary. Play, is an integral part of evaluation of most young children.

3. For children with behavioral problems, the evaluation should be:
   a. Psychoanalytical
   b. Behavioral
   c. Bio-psycho-social
   d. Neuropsychiatric

   Your answer is:

   Author's answer is: (c), bio-psycho-social. The other choices are too restrictive, limited, or biased in their approach. Children, whose behavior is the main source of complaint by parents or school authorities, may be suffering from various types of problems or illnesses. In order to understand the nature of the problem or illness and contributing factors, the evaluation should be comprehensive, encompassing the biological, psychological, and social aspects of the child.

4. Parents who bring their child for the child's first psychiatric evaluation, are usually:

   a. Very happy that the child eventually is getting a chance to be fully evaluated by a child psychiatrist

   b. Are anxious and worried

   c. Are hostile

   d. Most often are hoping that the doctor will prescribe an effective medicine the same day

   Your answer is:

Author's choice is: (b), "Are anxious and worried." Parents are usually worried about what and how serious the child's problem is, and what the psychiatrist may recommend. Bringing their child for the first time to a child psychiatrist is not usually a happy occasion for parents. They feel guilty and worried about the child's problems. They perceive the need for the child to be evaluated by the child psychiatrist, as an indication that the child's problems are not minor. Most parents would not want the child to be started on medicines, at least initially. They hope that the psychiatrist will tell them that the child's problems are not serious and can be dealt with by counseling, environmental manipulation, and related measures.

5. Children are more likely to talk openly when seen for an evaluation, if:
   a. The psychiatrist makes it very clear at the outset that they have to
   b. The psychiatrist offers to play with them
   c. The psychiatrist promises he or she will cure their problems
   d. They feel the clinician is genuinely concerned and interested in their welfare, and understands their situation

Your answer is:

Author's choice is: (d), "If they feel the clinician is genuinely concerned and interested in their welfare, and understands their situation." Demanding that they have to talk openly if they have to be helped, intimidates most children. Just involving the child in play activities, by itself, will not make children open up and talk about issues that are unpleasant for them. Making promises that are unrealistic, and cannot be kept, should be avoided. Children tend to talk more openly, if they feel the clinician is genuinely interested in their welfare, and understands their predicament.

6. Pre-requisites for the clinician conducting child psychiatric evaluation include:

a. Good knowledge of biological, psychological and social aspects of child development

b. Good knowledge of psychiatric problems that occur in childhood, and their signs and symptoms

c. Genuine interest and concern for children experiencing psychiatric problems

d. Capacity to tolerate provocative, distressing and annoying behavior

e. All of the above

Your answer is:

Author's choice is: (e), "All of the above." In order to do competent child psychiatric evaluations, one should have good knowledge of all aspects of child development. This includes the biological, psychological, and social aspects of development, and a good sense of the normal, delayed, and deviant aspects of development. Detailed and in depth knowledge of psychiatric problems and illnesses that manifest in children, and excellent capacity to detect their signs and symptoms are essential in conducting good evaluations of children. The evaluator should have genuine interest in children who suffer from psychiatric problems. Many psychiatrically ill, behaviorally disturbed, or developmentally disordered children needing evaluation could be distressing, annoying, or down right provocative in their behavior. A good evaluator should have capacity to understand and tolerate such situations without becoming distressed or annoyed unduly.

7. When interviewing the parents for the purpose of evaluating the child:
  a. It is essential to do a formal mental status examination of parents, because they are the primary caregivers
  b. Make an informal assessment of the mental functioning of the parents
  c. Focus on history gathering only, because that is what the parents are there for

Your answer is:

Author's choice is: (b), "Make an informal assessment of the mental functioning of the parents."

It is unwise and inappropriate to do a formal mental status examination of the parents when they bring their child for evaluation. However it is important to obtain a sense of the mental capacity and functioning of the parents. This is accomplished informally while obtaining information from them about the child and their concerns, and by observing the interactions between the parents, the parents and the child, and parents' interaction with the interviewer. History gathering is only one of the goals to be accomplished when the parents are seen.

8. The usual time required in conducting a child psychiatric evaluation and writing a report is:

a. ½ hour

b. ½—1 hour

c. 2-4 hours

d. 4-8 hours

Your answer is:

Author's choice is: (c), "2-4 hours."

Unless, a great deal of well-documented background information is already available, most evaluations and report writing together will take 2-4 hours. Interviewing the parents will require about an hour, and interviewing the child and observations during play will also take about an hour, in most cases. Writing a fairly comprehensive report can take anywhere from ½-1 hour. In addition, sufficient time has to be allotted to review material that may be available in the chart, such as, school and treatment reports, previous treatment records etc., prior to starting the evaluation. Sufficient time has to be reserved for the informing portion of the evaluation, in addition, during which the child and parents are apprised of the evaluator's findings and recommendations.

One hour or less is insufficient to do a good evaluation and produce a meaningful report. Four to eight hours is too long and unnecessary in most cases.

9. Once a child is found to be very hyperactive, impulsive, and his attention shifting from one object to another in rapid succession:

a. The diagnosis is pretty clear: it is ADHD

b. One can proceed with confidence to a Ritalin trial (after medical clearance)

c. One can proceed with a trial on one of the stimulants (after medical clearance)

d. The evaluation should take into account all conditions, which produce such a behavioral state

Your answer is:

Author's choice is: (d), "The evaluation should take into account all conditions that produce such a behavioral state".

A.D.H.D. is not the only condition that makes a child hyperactive, impulsive, and exhibit rapidly shifting attention from one stimulus or idea to another. A typical example is a child who is hypomanic or manic. Children in such states are among the most hyperactive and impulsive. Such children also shift from one object or idea to another in rapid succession. Many mentally retarded, and autistic children are also extremely hyperactive, impulsive, and exhibit poor capacity to remain attentive. All children who exhibit such characteristics require an open minded and thorough evaluation. Many clinicians unfortunately make up their mind that the child suffers from A.D.H.D., the moment the parents tell them that, the child's teacher has been complaining of such problems. The rest of the time spent in evaluation they consider to be perfunctory. This is one of the reasons why great many children end up carrying a diagnosis of A.D.H.D., often erroneously, throughout their childhood and even beyond.

10. If sufficient time is spend in evaluating a child:
    a. One can safely assume that the diagnoses arrived upon will be valid for the foreseeable future
    b. The diagnoses have to be considered preliminary and tentative

Your answer is:

Author's choice is: (b), "The diagnoses have to be considered preliminary and tentative"

Psychiatric diagnoses, in general, are at best approximations rather than being absolute facts at present. This is especially so in children. Compared to adults, children are in an accelerated state of development, which can change their behavior and symptomatology significantly from time to time. In addition, during the initial evaluation, the information available from the child, parents, school etc. are often incomplete. With more definitive information becoming available as time goes on and with further observations during treatment, the diagnostic understanding may change. At times parents, and children—especially adolescents—withhold crucial information during the initial phases of contact with the clinician, because of lack of trust, or fear that the clinician may consider them to be very ill or disturbed, or for a variety of other reasons.

11. When evaluating children or adolescents:
    a. Always interview the child first
    b. Always interview the parents first
    c. Always interview the adolescent first
    d. Make sure the child is allowed to play
    e. Take a flexible approach depending on the given situation

Your answer is:

Author's choice is:(e), "Take a flexible approach depending on the given situation".

With the evaluation of children and adolescents, the presenting problems and circumstances vary considerably. Though, often it is most appropriate to see the parents and child together for a brief introductory period, to get a sense of the presenting circumstances and explain to them the rough format of the evaluation process etc., followed by interviewing the parents, and then the child or adolescent, such a format may not be appropriate in all circumstances. For example, a young child may refuse to separate from the parents, and may have to be interviewed and observed in the presence of the parents. An adolescent may insist, that he or she has to be seen first, because of fear that the parents will distort information and prejudice the mind of the interviewer against him or her. These are only a few common examples of situations that call for the interviewer adjusting the format of the interview, to fit the needs of the presenting circumstances. It is not infrequent to run into a presenting problem or situation that would require great deal of flexibility on the part of the interviewer, as to how he or she may best conduct the evaluation. Such capacity to adapt the evaluation process to the needs of the presenting situation is a skill necessary for a good evaluator.

12. A child's guardian brings a child for an evaluation. The guardian is not a biological parent of the child. The guardian states that the child's parents occasionally visit the child. Before completing the evaluation:

a. Attempt should be made to interview the parents

b. It is futile to interview the parents because the child does not live with them

c. It is futile to interview the parents, because the guardian has already told you they are irresponsible people

d. It is futile to try to interview the parents, because such parents seldom keep their appointments

Your answer is:

Author's answer is: (a) "Attempt should be made to interview the parents". Psychiatric evaluation of children is seldom complete without interviewing the parents. The information that could be obtained by interviewing and observing the parents is of utmost importance, and in almost all cases will be highly revealing of the child and his or her problems. The unfortunate facts however are that, in today's circumstances many children who are brought for evaluation are not living with their parents, and the parents may not be available to be interviewed for one reason or another. However, reasonable attempts should be made to interview the parents as part of the evaluation of all children.

13. A foster parent brings a 15 year old for an evaluation with the complaints that the youngster steals, lies, is aggressive in school and elsewhere, is failing all his subjects, has been known to be drinking and smoking, and is becoming totally unmanageable in school and at home. The foster parent provided the only information available about the youngster's biological parents. The mother was reported to be a "drug addict and prostitute", and the father "is in jail for murder."

Given this information, you will:

    a. Primarily focus on conduct disorder as the child's problems

    b. Primarily focus on adjustment disorder as the most likely problem

    c. Primarily focus on depression as the underlying problem

    d. Primarily consider P.T.S.D. as the main problem

e. Remain open-minded, and consider all relevant issues and diagnostic possibilities

Your answer is:

Author's choice is: (e), "Remain open-minded, and consider all relevant issues and diagnostic possibilities"

Descriptions such as "prostitute", "drug addict", "in jail for murder" etc. do not mean that the people concerned have a particular type of problem or another. At best what can be surmised—if the information is at least somewhat correct—is that, the people concerned have had troubled lives. The nature of their problems could be highly varied. It is unwise to conclude that such descriptions automatically point to a particular type of problem or diagnosis. It is also unwise to conclude that, since the parents' history points to their having certain types of problems, the child also most likely suffers from such a problem. For example it is tempting to conclude prematurely that the parents suffer from severe personality disorders and the child from conduct disorder. So also, just because the child is in foster home, and the parents' history points to a troubled past, it is unwise to conclude that the child's problems are due to an adjustment reaction, or P.T.S.D—caused by separation from parents, exposure to traumatic events etc. Maintaining an open-mind, and considering all relevant issues and diagnostic possibilities is the best approach.

14. A mother brings her ten-year-old son who is suspended from school because of severe aggressive, explosive, and defiant behavior. The school guidance counselor has sent you a note stating that, the child has lately been showing severe behavior changes. At times he has also been found to be sad and depressed, and has revealed to her that at times he hears the "devil" urging him to do "bad things". When describing her son's problems and his reported hallucinations, his mother goes into inappropriate loud laughter, and makes statements such as, "He is crazy, he is a one-in-a-million crazy, I always knew he was crazy" etc. With this history, and observation regarding the mother, you will:

   a. Focus on thought disorder in the boy to confirm a diagnosis of schizophrenia

     b. Not give importance to what the mother says about the child after that, because she is uncaring and is disturbed herself

     c. Give serious consideration to the strong possibility that the mother is "Borderline"

     d. Will pay special attention to mother's informal mental status, and gently probe the topic of family history of psychiatric disorders

Your answer is:

Author's choice is: (d), "Will pay special attention to mother's informal mental status, and gently probe the topic of family history of psychiatric disorders"

Children reporting auditory hallucinations should not be automatically considered to be suffering from schizophrenia. In practice, many, if not most children, who report hallucinations such as the one described in this youngster, will be found to be suffering from a mood disorder, rather than a schizophrenic type of problem.

Even though the mother is acting inappropriately and may not be a well person herself, she may have a great deal of information about him, by the very fact she is his mother and has brought him for the evaluation. The best approach is to continue to gather history from her while keeping in mind that, she may not be very empathic to him, and that her understanding of his problems should not be accepted at face value

The term "borderline" is most often used today in a pejorative manner. It does not convey much useful meaning. Many people, termed "borderline" by clinicians who are often annoyed by their behavior, on closer scrutiny, are often found to be suffering from a major mental illness other than borderline personality disorder.

The mother's emotional state, and informal mental status should be ascertained in a careful manner. Parent's who behave in such manner, and make such utterances, are often found to be suffering from a major mental disorder—very often a mood disorder, such as bipolar disorder—that make them de-compensate and act inappropriately when faced with the frightening reality that their child or children are beginning to exhibit signs of a mental illness. It is quite common to come across such parents when dealing with children who exhibit signs of a major mental illness. Such parents require a very supportive and empathic approach.

15. A mother brings her nine-year-old son for an evaluation. He is hyperactive, impulsive, aggressive, quick to anger—with an explosive temperament, and has become very difficult to manage in school and at home. The school authorities want to place him in special education because of his behavior problems. Mother states, that his problems started after the city wrongly accused her of child abuse, and placed him in a foster home, from the time he was seven until about a year back. She is considering suing the city. Given this information you will:

a. Completely believe the mother's statements, and direct your inquiries to validate a diagnosis of Adjustment Disorder

b. Channel your enquiries to validate a diagnosis of P.T.S.D.

c. Disbelieve the mother because the child is showing classical features of A.D.H.D

d. Disbelieve the mother, since she will distort facts to obtain compensation from the city

e. Continue to obtain details of past history and development, and make arrangements to get school reports of the past several years

Your answer is:

Author's choice is: (d) "Will continue to obtain details of past history and development…past several years"

History, such as the one given by this mother is very commonly encountered when evaluating children, especially in clinic settings. Though their intentions may be quite honest, parents often may not be correct in their perception or memory of when a child's problems surfaced. This is understandable, since behavior problems of children often do not surface abruptly, but rather develop in a slow and uneven manner beginning in early childhood, eventually reaching crisis proportions as years go by. Often, parents give a history of a traumatic event—a foster home placement could be traumatic to both the child and parents—as having been the precipitant for the child's problems. This may, or may not be true. What is needed is an open-minded approach, clarifying details of past history, and obtaining documentation as to the development of the problems. School records of the past few years will be very useful for such purposes.

16. A six-year-old, cute-looking-girl is brought in for evaluation. Her teacher has warned that the child may not be promoted this year because of lack of academic progress. Parents' state that the child is "very smart", but is "lazy". The child was born premature, weighing four pounds. You will pay special attention to:

a. Developmental history

b. Speech and language capacities

c. Capacity to do paper and pencil tasks appropriate for age

d. Parents' understanding and attitude toward the child's strengths and weaknesses

e. All of the above

Your answer is:

Author's choice is: (e) "All of the above"

Learning disabilities and cognitive deficiencies are common in children born prematurely, and of low birth weight. Delays or deviations in development are common in such children. Academic problems surface in some such children during the early grades. Parents often are reluctant to admit, or do not perceive their child may be experiencing such difficulties. To acknowledge that their child may have such deficiencies is upsetting to most parents. Many children, who have learning disabilities, or mild cognitive deficiencies, appear and behave in a "normal" manner during early childhood, which the parents interpret to mean that the child has normal or average capacities at least, but is not achieving academically because of laziness.

17. A mother brings in her sixteen-year-old daughter for an evaluation The mother states that her daughter was arrested twice in the recent past for assault and drug possession. Mother has been a high school teacher for the past several years. She states, that she is devastated by her daughter's behavior. Lately her daughter has been running away from home, and engaging in dangerous behavior with a group of youngsters who have similar behavior problems. A few days back she made superficial cuts on her wrist, and started sobbing when the mother asked her what was troubling her. You note, that the girl has dyed her hair purple and is wearing an assortment of earrings and

nose-rings. She appears tired and disheveled. During her evaluation you will pay special attention to:

a. Getting the girls opinion as to what is happening to her, and her mental status

b. Detailed gathering of history from the child and her mother, including pertinent symptomatology, sleep patterns etc.

c. Detailed information about the father

d. Family history of psychiatric disorders

e. All of the above

Your answer is:

The author's choice is: (e), "All of the above."

The problems presented by this sixteen-year-old are commonly encountered in clinical practice, and often present challenges in ascertaining the nature of the problem, appropriate diagnosis, and providing effective treatment. Detailed history gathering, elucidating the symptomatology—especially symptomatology that will help distinguish between conduct disorder and a mood disorder such as bipolar disorder—are essential when evaluating such children. Information about the father and family history of psychiatric disorders are crucial in arriving upon proper diagnosis in such children. If at all possible, the father should be seen before completing the evaluation. Inability or refusal to sleep often points to a mood disorder rather than conduct disorder. The fact that the youngster was found distressed, and engaged in wrist cutting should also alert the clinician to search for possible underlying mood disorder. Often, there is a tendency to quickly dismiss such youngsters as just exhibiting conduct disorder—a grave mistake.

18. A mother has brought her fifteen-year-old son for a re-evaluation. From the time he was in first grade, he has received stimulant medicines and psychotherapy from the same clinic. Presently, you are beginning work as the new child psychiatrist for the clinic. The youngster is known to be "very intelligent" (I.Q. 136), but is failing almost all subjects. His behavior has become unmanageable in school and very difficult at home. He was suspended several times recently, and the school authorities are planning to "kick him out". His past records reveal that he has been given a diagnosis of A.D.H.D. and oppositional defiant disorder by the psychiatrists

who evaluated him. There is an occasional mention in teachers' and therapists' notes that he appeared depressed. Recently, conduct disorder was added as an additional diagnosis, and placement in a residential treatment center was recommended. On reviewing his chart, you note, that his behavior has been more problematic periodically, reaching crisis proportions at times. There are strong indications from the history that he may be suffering from bipolar disorder. You inquire about family history of psychiatric problems. Parents have been divorced for the past five years. Mother states that she never had reasons to seek psychiatric treatment. As far as she knows, his father also was never in treatment. Such problems do not "run" in their families, she states.

Following such statements by the mother, you will:

a. Move on to other relevant topics

b. Ask the mother about her sleep patterns

c. Gently ask the mother to give a description of the personality functioning of both parents

d. Question the mother why they got divorced if they didn't have problems

Your answer is:

Author's choice is: (c), "Gently ask the mother to give a description of the personality functioning of both parents."

A statement, that a parent or parents have never been in psychiatric treatment, or that one of the parents had no reason to seek psychiatric treatment, by itself, does not mean that the parent or parents, have not experienced significant psychiatric problems. The topic needs further, gentle and supportive exploration. However a confrontational and inappropriate question such as the one in choice (d), about parental divorce, or an immediate move to elicit possible symptomatology in the mother that may support your suspicions, as in choice (b), are inappropriate and unwise.

19. You are continuing the evaluation of the fifteen-year-old male youngster mentioned in the previous question (18). His mother states, that his father had an explosive temper, and was at times physically abusive. He had difficulty keeping jobs, in spite of being very intelligent and having a degree from a highly prestigious

institution. He has a gambling problem, drinks excessively at times, and is a "womanizer", she says—reasons why she divorced him. He is now living with another woman. He sees the boy occasionally, but often breaks promises he makes to him. She thinks, her son's problems are due to the father's rejecting and uncaring attitude.

Given this information you will:

    a. Make further inquiries about the father, especially if she knows of any tendency for him to go through periods of depression

    b. Inquire if she knows much about father's own parents, and siblings if any, and ask her to describe them and their personalities

    c. Make sure to ask the youngster about his father, and his relationship to him

    d. All of the above

Your answer is:

Author's choice is: (d), all of the above

The father's history is highly indicative of a person who very likely suffers from a mood disorder—such as bipolar disorder. Many such people go through a lifetime of suffering and troubled behavior, without ever being identified as suffering from such illness. Many will refuse treatment even if they are advised, that such treatment may make their life more manageable. Detailed inquiry about their life and functioning, aimed at clarifying patterns of behavior and symptomatology that is highly indicative of such mood disorders is necessary, in arriving upon proper conclusions about the behavior and symptomatology of the type of youngster we are presently concerned about. Additional clarification can often be obtained by inquiries regarding the personality and functioning of the youngster's grandparents and other first and second-degree relatives. Such inquiries in a concerned and supportive manner is essential with all children suspected to be possibly suffering from an illness such as bipolar disorder, which often goes unrecognized all through their lives.

20. A mother brings her ten-year-old son for an evaluation. He is reported to be overactive, disruptive and aggressive in school. He poses similar problems at home also, but his mother says she knows how to manage him. She blames the teachers for his school problems. They don't know how to give him the attention and understanding he

deserves, she states. They blame her son when other children are at fault. She threatens to sue. Mother is emotionally volatile, verbally explosive, and uses great deal of profanity when expressing her opinion and concerns. You get the sense that the mother is not an emotionally well person, and probably suffers from a significant psychiatric illness. When enquired about possible family history of psychiatric problems, she flatly denies any such problems among any of the child's close relatives. She exhibits obvious irritation and annoyance at your questioning her about such matters. Now you will:

a. Tell her that you are an expert in psychiatric problems, and as such, do not believe she is telling the truth

b. Tell her that in your opinion she suffers from a mental illness, hoping this will make her be more honest

c. Move on to other topics, as it is important to maintain rapport and unwise to confront such, possible denial, in the present situation

Your answer is:

Author's choice is: (c), "Move on to other topics…Situation."

This mother's demeanor, utterances and volatility strongly suggest that she may indeed have significant emotional problems—if not, even a major psychiatric illness. It is also quite likely that, she and her son may be unfortunately suffering from similar type of illness. However inquiry about psychiatric problems in family members is a very sensitive topic, and should be dealt with in a very cautious, sensitive, and supportive manner only. Parents often deny such problems, because of fear that their child may be misunderstood, or automatically be thought of as suffering from the type of problem or illness his biological relatives suffer from. It is important to maintain rapport with the parents during the evaluation, and also not make them unduly upset. If a parent denies a history of emotional or psychiatric problems in themselves or other family members, even though there may be some evidence to the contrary, confronting them about it during the evaluation is inappropriate and unwise. It is most appropriate to move on to other topics. During future contacts with the parents, opportunity may arise to re-visit the topic again, when the parents feel more trusting and ready to be open about it.

21. You see a seven-year-old girl for an evaluation. She talks spontaneously and openly, and answers your questions appropriately, providing relevant information. Since the interview is going smoothly you do not introduce the child to play activities.

   a. The interview is incomplete because the child has not been observed in play.

   b. It was a mistake not to have interrupted the interview to find enough time for play

   c. Though play is very useful in the evaluation of young children, it is not absolutely essential for all children and circumstances

Your answer is:

Author's choice is: (c), "Though play is very useful…Circumstances."

The purpose of the interview is to obtain as much information about the child that is relevant for the evaluation. Since children often have difficulty providing sufficient information about them and their concerns by face-to-face verbal interchange only, play is often a very useful tool to gather such information by indirect means. This does not mean that play is absolutely essential to complete an evaluation with all children and in all circumstances. Occasionally one comes across young children who can provide sufficient meaningful information in a face-to-face interview. There are also circumstances in which introducing a child to play may not always be appropriate—for example a child who has just experienced a catastrophic loss, is sad and overwhelmed by it, and is being evaluated in that connection.

22. A ten-year-old boy who has carried a diagnosis of autism since he was a toddler, and whose intelligence is in the severely retarded range, is brought in for an evaluation. He attends a special educational program for such children. He is non-verbal and has not been toilet trained. His parents state that he has been very hyperactive and impulsive all his life. He often slept poorly. He has been given Ritalin to address hyperactivity and related problems, but it had not been found to be effective. The medicine may have even made him worse at times, the parents state. During the past two weeks the child has become much more hyperactive and agitated. He has not slept at all the last two days, and has been

constantly running, climbing on objects without concern for danger, and has been making screaming and howling noises almost non-stop. He doesn't seem to tire they say, though they are afraid he could just collapse from such non-stop activity. Nobody in the house can rest because of his behavior. They are totally exhausted, and at their "wits end", the parents say.

a. In the evaluation of this child it is most important to observe for evidence of stereotypies to confirm the diagnosis of autism.

b. In the evaluation of the child it is most important to obtain a detailed family history, to ascertain whether other close relatives suffered from autism or mental retardation.

c. It is most important to obtain details of the child's behavior problems through the years, especially any waxing and waning patterns in their intensity, and obtain a family history of psychiatric disorders.

Your answer is:

Author's choice is: (c), "It is most important to obtain details of the child's behavior problems…family history of psychiatric disorders."

In evaluating a child who is exhibiting acute, distressing, and dangerous symptomatology as this child is, it is most important that the evaluation address those problems primarily. The fact, that this child is significantly mentally retarded and has autistic features, is already known and would be easily evident. Confirming such facts once more, by itself, will not address the current presenting problems, which are causing extreme distress to the child and parents. Though many autistic, and mentally retarded children exhibit hyperactivity, impulsivity, and related problems, what this child has been experiencing and exhibiting recently, cannot be explained by a diagnosis of autism or mental retardation alone. The acute worsening of his behavior, especially the non-stop excited and agitated behavior, and the history that he has not slept for days, points most probably to his suffering from a mental illness—apart from autism and mental retardation. Only details of his behavior problems as they occurred through the years, possible remissions and exacerbations, cyclical patterns if any, and family history of psychiatric disorders if any—and the nature of the illness or illnesses if they are present—will clarify the nature of this child's problems. When evaluating autistic or mentally retarded children with severe behavior problems, always keep in mind that such a child has at least an equal chance to suffer from an additional, serious mental illness, compared to youngsters who are not autistic or mentally retarded.

23. A five-year-old child refuses to enter the office with or without his parents. When you try to persuade him to come into the office, he cries, clings to his parents, and throws a severe temper tantrum. Given this situation:

a. It is quite clear the child cannot be effectively evaluated in the outpatient setting

b. It is quite clear separation anxiety disorder is the child's main problem

c. You try to allay the child's fears and engage him or her in play activities, by bringing play materials to him in the waiting area and continue your observations.

Your answer is:

Author's choice is: (c), "You try to allay the child's fears…continue your observations."

Fear and resistance, as exhibited by this child, is quite common in many such young children when they are brought for an evaluation. Often they equate such visits with painful procedures such as injections, blood drawing etc. Just because a young child is exhibiting separation problems and fear, it does not mean that separation anxiety disorder is the child's main problem. Attempts could be made to observe the child in the waiting area itself, by allaying his or her fears with efforts as mentioned in choice (c). At times such children may require more than one visit to complete an evaluation adequately. Do not forget that all of a child's behavior—including uncooperative behavior—is revealing of the child and his or her problems.

24. At the end of an evaluation, when informing the parents and child of the relevant findings and recommendations, the most important thing to keep in mind is:

    a. The clinician should be very thorough in explaining how the diagnosis was arrived upon

    b. Be very honest to the child, and do not tell the parents anything that one is not prepared to tell the child

    c. Be supportive

Your answer is:

Author's choice is: (c), "Be supportive."

Parents and children are almost always apprehensive about how serious the problems may be and what remedies may be recommended. The feedback given after an evaluation should be in lay terms the child and parents can easily understand. Giving a child an official diagnosis for his problems is often unnecessary, if not inappropriate, except in situations where using such terms could help the child understand his problems better and feel that the nature of his suffering or problems is not unusual or mysterious. Most often, what is more useful for the parents and child to know is the nature of the child's problems and what could be done about it. If the parents ask for an official diagnosis, or if it is relevant in helping them understand the nature of the child's problems, it is appropriate to give them specific diagnostic terms and explain to them what the terms mean. At times it may be useful or necessary to discuss with the parents or an adolescent why the clinician arrived upon such a conclusion.

In all circumstances when informing the child, and parents, of the clinician's findings, be supportive. This is the most important thing to keep in mind throughout the evaluation, and especially in the informing session.

Afterword

As mentioned in the beginning, the psychiatric evaluation of children as it stands today is at a very incomplete and imprecise state. There is great hope that the revolution in molecular biology, genetics, functional brain imaging, and related endeavors underway will soon give it a precision long hoped for, and with it our capacity to institute vastly improved and precise, if not curative, treatment measures. The method of evaluating the child and his problems is bound to undergo changes with the scientific advances, but the essential interpersonal element in doing good evaluations will continue to play the crucial role, as it does presently.

In the psychiatric evaluation of the child, the concerned, sensitive clinician adapts and improvises on the guidelines, in his or her own unique style, for the benefit of the child and the family, and in furthering our understanding of children and their families in distress, This core ingredient remains crucial today and will remain so for the future to come.

About the Author

Dr. George Isaac, is a Child Psychiatrist who has practiced and taught Child and Adult Psychiatry in the United States, Canada, and India during the past three decades. He presently lives and works in New York City.

Made in United States
North Haven, CT
29 August 2023